RO 11·10

0 6 NOV 2015

2 4 JUL 2017

CW00371564

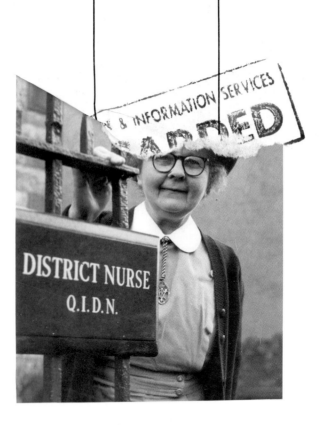

LD 4235242 8

Published in Great Britain in 2010 by Shire Publications
Ltd, Midland House, West Way, Botley, Oxford OX2 0PH,
United Kingdom.

44-02 23rd Street, Suite 219, Long Island City, NY 11101,
USA.

E-mail: shire@shirebooks.co.uk   www.shirebooks.co.uk

© 2010 Susan Cohen.

All rights reserved. Apart from any fair dealing for the
purpose of private study, research, criticism or review, as
permitted under the Copyright, Designs and Patents Act,
1988, no part of this publication may be reproduced,
stored in a retrieval system, or transmitted in any form or
by any means, electronic, electrical, chemical, mechanical,
optical, photocopying, recording or otherwise, without the
prior written permission of the copyright owner.
Enquiries should be addressed to the Publishers.

Every attempt has been made by the Publishers to secure
the appropriate permissions for materials reproduced in
this book. If there has been any oversight we will be happy
to rectify the situation and a written submission should be
made to the Publishers.

A CIP catalogue record for this book is available from the
British Library.

Shire Library no. 609.   ISBN-13: 978 0 74780 808 4

Susan Cohen has asserted her right under the Copyright,
Designs and Patents Act, 1988, to be identified as the
author of this book.

Designed by Tony Truscott Designs, Sussex, UK
and typeset in Perpetua and Gill Sans.

Printed in China through Worldprint Ltd.

**LEEDS LIBRARIES AND
INFORMATION SERVICE**

LD 4235242 8	
HJ	08-Nov-2010
610.7 3	£6.99
S035179	

COVER IMAGE
District Nurse Jeal with the Medical Officer at an infant
welfare clinic, 1950s.

TITLE PAGE IMAGE
A Queen's Nurse leaving her house in Edinburgh in the
1950s.

CONTENTS PAGE IMAGE
Eight of the twenty-one district nurses employed by
Berkshire County Council with new Mini Minors, which
they had recently exchanged for their ten-year-old cars
(*District Nursing*, June 1960).

ACKNOWLEDGEMENTS
I would like to thank the Queen's Nursing Institute, and
specifically Professor Rosemary Cook, CBE, Director,
and Matthew Bradby, Marketing and Communications
Manager, for the help they have given me and for allowing
me to use illustrations from the QNI archive. My thanks
also to Sue Machell for giving permision for me to
reproduce unpublished cartoons of her grandmother,
District Nurse Elsie Malcolm, drawn by a patient in
Newcastle in the 1920s.

All illustrations are reproduced by courtesy of the Queen's
Nursing Institute, except for the following:

Edinburgh Evening News, title page; Imperial War Museum,
page 30; A. J. Knowler, page 48; Liverpool Record Office,
pages 8, 9, 10, 12 (bottom), 19 and 26 (bottom);
Sue Machell, pages 26 (top right) and 28 (bottom);
Portsmouth City Libraries, page 12 (top); Barnet Saidman
(QNI), pages 42 and 52; *Western Morning News*, 44.

For the images on pages 3, 22, 48 (bottom) and 53, every
effort has been made to trace copyright holders, and the
author and the Queen's Nursing Institute would be
grateful for any information which might help trace those
whose addresses are not known.

Several of the pictures in this book have been taken from
original printed material and any deficiencies in picture
quality are a result of this.

Shire Publications is supporting the Woodland Trust, the UK's leading woodland conservation charity, by funding the dedication of trees.

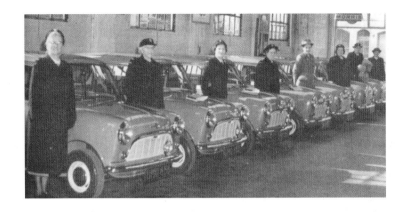

CONTENTS

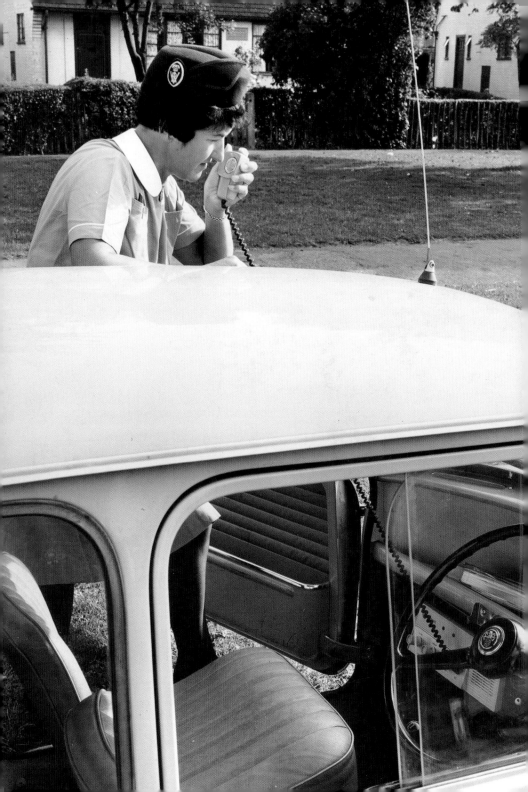

INTRODUCTION

SICK PEOPLE have been nursed at home for centuries, but before the advent of professionally trained nurses and district nurses in Britain in the late nineteenth century the poor had few options open to them. They either had to rely upon the generosity of untrained family members and neighbours to care for them in times of sickness, or call upon either of the twin pillars of social policy, the Poor Law and charity. Up until 1834 most Poor Law relief was given as 'outdoor', so the recipients of help did not have to enter the dreaded workhouse. Although many parishes did employ a so-called nurse, her duties were quite unclear and had little to do with administering medical care, nor was she qualified in any way. Nurse Philpot in Bath was one such person; according to Mary Stocks, her activities included dispensing senna and salts, and she was allowed money for brimstone and treacle. The alternative was services provided by charitable organisations, especially those of a religious nature, such as the Society of Protestant Sisters of Charity, the Quakers and the Anglican Oxford Movement, but the overall picture was one of incompetence and ignorance.

Nursing care, such as it was, was very basic, administered by women who were often regarded as no better than domestic servants. Charles Dickens graphically characterised the early Victorian nurse in *Martin Chuzzlewit* in 1844. His domiciliary nurse, the 'handywoman' Sairy (Sarah) Gamp, was 'the female functionary, a nurse, a watcher', who was more often than not drunk, whilst her hospital counterpart, Betsy Prig, had very little training and was given no responsibility.

In 1850s Britain nursing was an occupation in desperate need of reform, but thanks to Florence Nightingale's efforts, and the royalties from her book *Notes on Nursing*, first published in 1859, the Nightingale School of Nursing was established at St Thomas's Infirmary (now St Thomas's Hospital) and the profession of nursing was born. Meanwhile, the healthcare of the poorest in society remained neglected, and such patients were reliant on untrained people to meet their medical needs. But this was about to change with the establishment of a new type of nurse.

Opposite:
A district nurse sending a message from her car by radio telephone in the early 1970s.

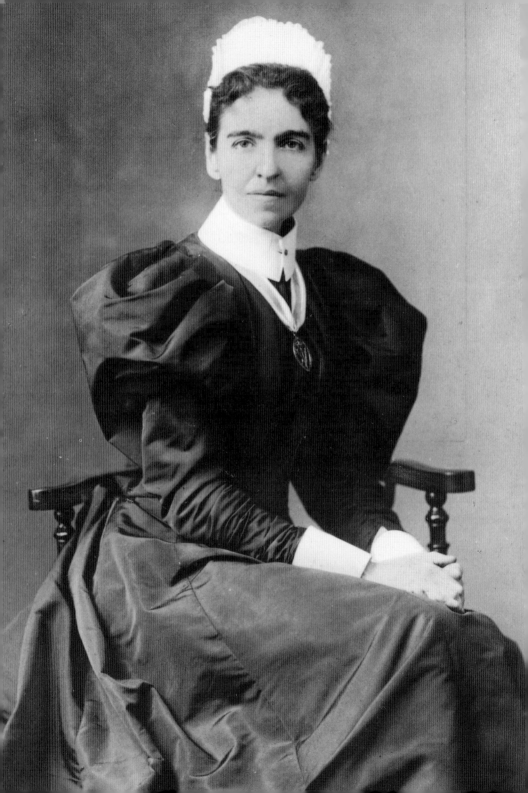

THE EARLY YEARS

THE STORY of how the district nurse came to be a welcome, trusted and caring member of the community, providing professional nursing care and support in homes throughout the British Isles, began in the mid-nineteenth century. By that time many well-meaning individuals had made efforts to make skilled nursing available to the poor in their own homes, for example Elizabeth Fry, who established the Institution of Nursing Sisters at 4 Devonshire Square, Bishopsgate, London, in 1845. Three years later another scheme to provide professionally trained nurses was set up by the Society of St John's House, whose mission had a religious and moral dimension.

But it was William Rathbone, a Liverpool philanthropist, who was responsible for bringing about a revolution in district nursing. In 1859 he discovered that Liverpool's sick poor lacked any healthcare, so he decided to try an experiment for three months: he engaged Mary Robinson, a trained nurse who had tended his late wife, to visit the sick poor in their homes and to 'teach the rules of health and comfort'. The trial almost failed, for, within weeks, Miss Robinson was overwhelmed by the amount of misery she encountered, and begged to be released from the post. Fortunately, not only was she persuaded to stay, but before long she asked to remain permanently. This gave a delighted William Rathbone the impetus to extend the service and employ more nurses, but he found it impossible to find what he described as 'women with the necessary experience and good character to be entrusted with the work'. He consulted Florence Nightingale, whom he considered 'in matters of nursing, to be my Pope', and through their combined efforts – his philanthropy and her expertise – a new training school and home for nurses, including district nurses, was built and opened at the Liverpool Royal Infirmary in 1863. With William Rathbone's concept of a hospital-trained district nurse now established, eighteen 'districts' of manageable size were created across the city, and a system of local nursing associations was inaugurated. By 1905 the whole of the city was within the reach of a nurse and, as a booklet published by the Liverpool Institute reported, 'there is no street, alley, court or cellar where their services may not be obtained'.

Opposite:
Dame Rosalind Paget (1855–1948) was a trained nurse. She was 1st Queens Nurse and Inspector, 1890–91. Her Uncle was William Rathbone.

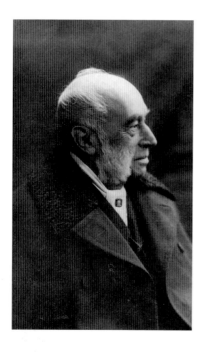

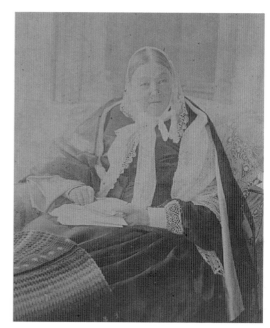

Above: William Rathbone, who inaugurated the idea of employing trained nurses to attend to the health needs of poor people in their own homes in Liverpool.

Above right: Florence Nightingale, 1895. She worked with William Rathbone to establish the concept of district nursing.

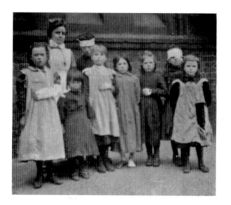

A district nurse with some of her patients in Liverpool, c. 1905.

District nurses were soon at work in other industrial towns and cities as the Liverpool model was gradually adopted elsewhere, including Manchester (1864), Derby (1865) and Leicester (1867). The situation was different in London, which had its own schemes for providing nursing care. A small group of 'Biblewomen nurses' were introduced in the deprived district of Seven Dials in 1868 by Mrs Ranyard, an ardent supporter of the British and Foreign Bible Society. Poorly trained, many of her working-class 'Biblewomen' received no more than three months' training at Guy's Hospital, and divided their work between proselytising and patching up their poor patients. Within six years there were forty-eight Ranyard district nurses working in the capital, alongside seven private nurses engaged by another organisation, the East London Nursing Society, who tended the sick poor in their own homes in the local districts of Bromley-by-Bow, Poplar and St Philips, and Stepney Way. But even the combined efforts of fifty-five district nurses barely scratched the surface of need. Besides this, the standard of care offered to the poor was pitifully inadequate, prompting an investigation into the provision of district nursing in London. In 1875, with more help and advice from William Rathbone, the Metropolitan and National Association for Providing Trained Nurses for the Sick Poor (MNA) was set up in Bloomsbury Square, London, with its own Central Home and Training School, setting the standard for training in the capital.

Innovation was one thing, but funding this revolutionary enterprise was quite another. Help came unexpectedly from Queen Victoria, who was celebrating her Golden Jubilee in 1887. There was an excess of £70,000 available from the Women's Jubilee Offering, and the Queen proposed that the money be made available for the welfare of nurses, a cause that was very dear to her heart. The decision to establish a nationwide consolidated district

A typical Liverpool court, c. 1905. The inhabitants of such deprivation benefited greatly from the services of a district nurse.

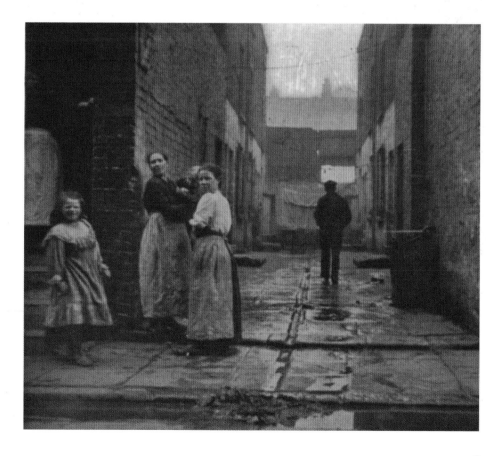

nursing organisation embodied all of William Rathbone's and Florence Nightingale's cherished ideals, the keynote being professional training, and so the Queen Victoria Jubilee Institute for Nurses (QVJIN) was inaugurated under Royal Charter in 1889.

The organisation wasted no time in embarking upon a national system of training, inspection and affiliation. The *Queen's Nurses' Magazine* (*QNM*), launched in 1904, became the best source of information on the activities of the district nursing movement and soon set out the entry requirements for candidates.

To apply for the Queen's approval and be admitted to the Queen's Roll, an applicant needed a minimum of two years' hospital experience, followed by six months of district training and the passing of an examination. State Registration became a prerequisite for acceptance for Queen's training once it was placed on the statute book in 1919, and by 1928 the hospital practice requirement had been increased to three years. The appointment of Superintendents, whose job was to undertake regular inspections, guaranteed that high standards of nursing were maintained and had the added benefit of enabling district nurses, wherever they were located, to be part of what *Nursing Notes* described in June 1903 as 'this great central organization'.

The intention of affiliation was much the same; the majority of District Nursing Associations (DNAs), whose job was to provide a trained nurse or nurses for the benefit of local people, regardless of individual financial

Nurses leaving the Liverpool Central Home to visit their patients, c. 1905.

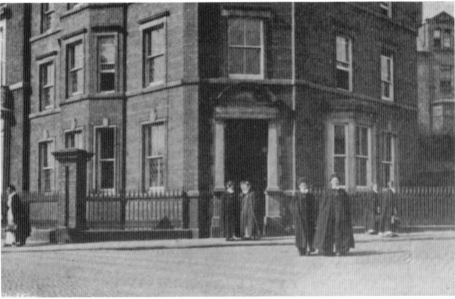

circumstances, did, like Portsmouth, become part of the Institute. A few, however, such as the Bristol and Clifton Nurses' Society, founded in 1881, and the Council of District Nursing for the City of Newcastle, established in 1883, chose to remain independent right up to the mid-1940s. Nevertheless, the same high training standards were maintained, and their district nurses provided a similar service to patients as the Queen's Nurses. Until the introduction of the National Health Service in 1948, all district nurses' wages and living expenses were paid by their local association. This included the provision of accommodation, and in the early years the district nurse working in a large town was obliged to live in a nurses' home, under the charge of a trained superintendent approved by the council, whilst those in rural areas were often put up in lodgings. Up to the end of the Second World War, most district nurses were unmarried, and DNAs often purchased private houses that they converted to provide accommodation, equipment and treatment facilities for their staff. In August 1930, Yardley in Birmingham established its fifth nurses' home, while in 1937 the home in Guildford, Surrey, even included a labour ward. Things were quite different by the mid-1950s, for the majority of district nurses were married women who lived at home and worked from 8.30 a.m. to 5.30 p.m.

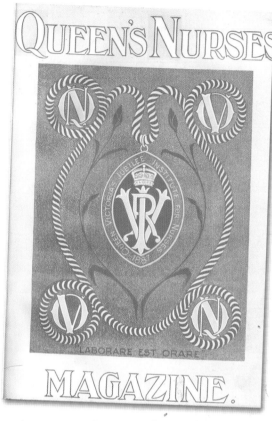

The front cover of the *Queen's Nurses' Magazine*, 30 April 1909.

Raising money was a constant challenge for the DNAs, who tapped a variety of sources including charitable donations, fund-raising events, house-to-house collections, gifts and voluntary subscriptions, many of which involved the Superintendent and her nurses. When the 1911 National Insurance Act was introduced, it provided an attractive way of paying for home nursing by way of provident schemes. In Leicester in 1929, for example, the secretary of the local association advised charging one penny a fortnight to subscribers, while those who were not subscribers would be charged 1s 6d for each visit. With 60,000 workers subscribing, more than 80,000 home visits were made by nurses in the city that year; the income rose

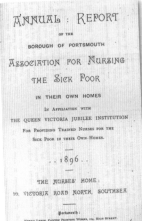

ANNUAL : REPORT
OF THE
BOROUGH OF PORTSMOUTH
Association for Nursing
THE Sick Poor
IN THEIR OWN HOMES
IN AFFILIATION WITH
THE QUEEN VICTORIA JUBILEE INSTITUTION
FOR PROVIDING TRAINED NURSES FOR THE
SICK POOR IN THEIR OWN HOMES.

.. 1896 ..

THE NURSES' HOME:
99, VICTORIA ROAD NORTH, SOUTHSEA

Above: Title page
of the Annual
Report for 1896
of the Borough
of Portsmouth
Victoria
Association
for Nursing
the Sick Poor.

from £3,000 to £9,000 per year, and the number of nurses employed increased from eighteen to thirty.

Queen Victoria was very proud of her nurses and in 1896 invited all 539 on the Queen's Roll to visit Windsor. Nearly four hundred of them accepted, and the women, decked out in their uniforms, were transported by special train from London. Mary Stocks described how

Lunch was provided in a marquee ... At 5 o'clock, they were assembled in the Park for inspection by the Queen, who, in her speech, said 'I am very pleased to see my nurses here today, to hear of the good work they are doing and I am sure will continue to do.'

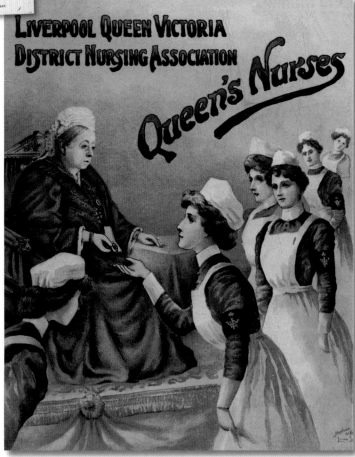

Right:
Queen Victoria
distributing badges
to Queen's Nurses
of the Liverpool
Queen Victoria
District Nursing
Association,
c. 1897.

12

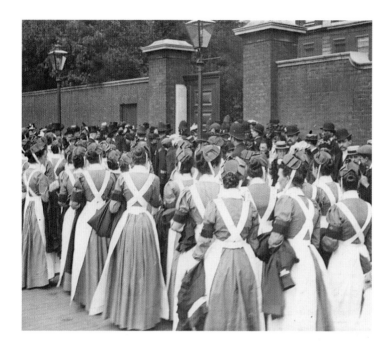

Queen's Nurses waiting to enter Buckingham Palace, 1901. Queen Victoria established a tradition of inviting nurses to the Palace, which continued in subsequent reigns.

That it was able to do so owed much to the Queen's generosity, for when she celebrated her Diamond Jubilee in 1897 a further royal endowment of £84,000 was made to the QVJIN. Over the decades district nurses on the Queen's Roll were regularly invited to meet their royal patrons at venues including Windsor Castle, Buckingham Palace, St James's Palace and Holyrood House, Scotland.

Queen's Nurses being presented to the royal entourage at Holyrood House, Edinburgh, in 1934.

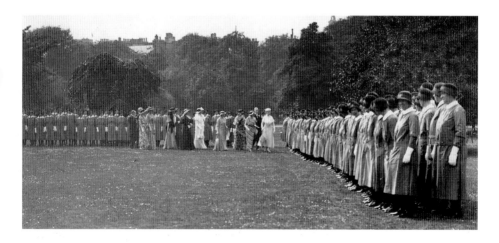

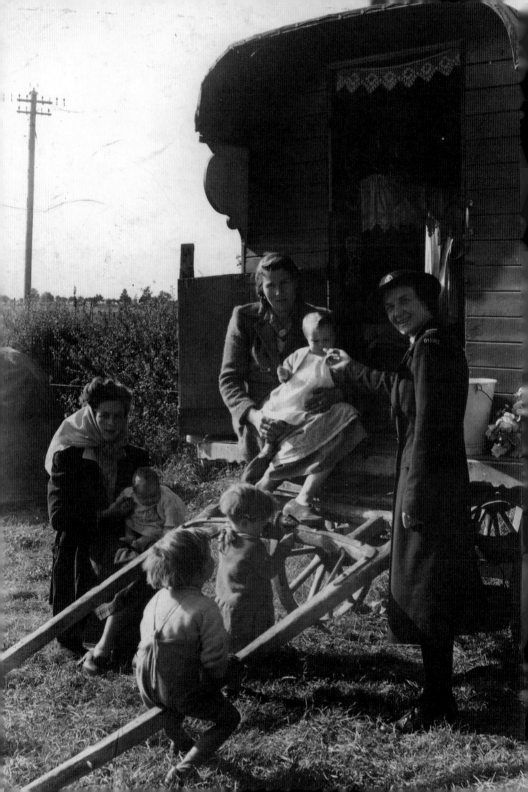

THE GROWTH OF DISTRICT NURSING

WITH THE IMPETUS for new associations established, it was not long before Wales, Scotland and Ireland followed suit and responded to the desperate nursing needs of their sick poor. Wales presented a special problem, as Welsh-speaking district nurses were required in many parts of the country. By the end of 1892 there were, according to Mary Stocks, seven DNAs operating in Wales, a number which steadily increased until the establishment of the National Health Service in 1948. Local communities in the mining valleys of South Wales, where industrial injuries were commonplace, were particularly wary of 'strangers' and the district nurse was often viewed with suspicion until her qualifications and abilities were accepted.

In Scotland, the Glasgow Sick and Poor Private Nursing Association was initiated by Mrs Mary Higginbotham in 1875, and the Queen's Nursing Institute Scotland (QNIS) was founded in Edinburgh in the same year, with Queen Victoria's daughter, Princess Louise, Marchioness of Lorne, appointed president. The Glasgow association became affiliated to the QVJIN in 1889 and before long had fourteen district nurses in training. Two district nurses employed by the Clydebank district, set up in 1907, had their wages paid for by two local firms, the sewing-machine manufacturers Singer and John Brown's shipyards. County associations were formed in Ayrshire, Fife and Lothian in 1914, and at the same time a scheme was inaugurated whereby district nurses were supplied to the Highlands and Islands Medical Service, serving the isolated island communities. Whether the inhabitants of St Kilda, one of the remotest locations in the Outer Hebrides, were all in good health, as the district nurse maintained in April 1918, is questionable, since they were, according to her, too busy spinning to complain. The newly appointed district nurse on the island of Burra in Shetland also had a busy first year in 1918, dealing with epidemics of chicken-pox and many cases of blood poisoning from fish-hooks, as well as fourteen maternity cases. By 1961 there were 1,068 district nurses employed by 586 Scottish DNAs, with rural duties for the 'island' nurses still a combination of nursing, midwifery and health visiting.

Opposite:
A district nurse visiting a gipsy caravan in the 1940s.

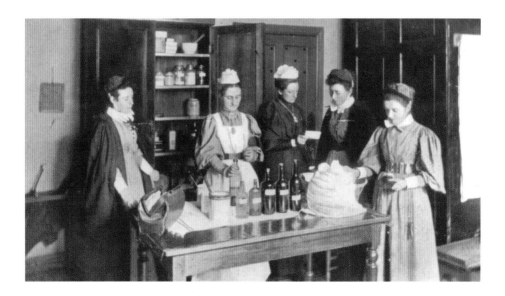

Scottish district nurses getting ready to go out into the district, c. 1900.

That district nurses began to attend the poor in Ireland owed much to William Rathbone, who devoted considerable time and money to promoting a service in Dublin, doing much to overcome sectarian divisions. St Patrick's Home for District Nurses was founded in Dublin by Lady Plunkett in 1876, but it was not until 1903 that Lady Dudley, the wife of the Lord Lieutenant, set up her 'Fund for District Nurses'. By March 1904 her appeals for financial support had raised enough money to 'establish and endow eight Jubilee nurses', who worked in the very poorest parts of Ireland, and in April 1908 the *QNM* reported that the committee had arranged to send nurses to Derrybeg, County Donegal, and Kiltimagh, County Mayo. The district nurse in Bangor, County Down, was credited with having done more to raise the standard of health and hygiene than an army of sanitary inspectors, because she entered the house to give much-needed help, while the inspector's visits were often regarded with suspicion and distrust. Even though eleven more district nurses had been endowed within eighteen months, they could only touch the tip of the iceberg: the unfulfilled demand for nursing care was huge, as an urgent appeal from the parish priest in the Aran Isles, published in the *QNM* in August 1905, made clear:

> On this island of Innishman we have a population of over 2,500 souls with only, I might say, fresh air and God's providence to tend them. No nursing and no care. At the present moment there are numerous cases of scarlatina. The Medical Officer is sick and not a word or suggestion as to treatment save only the poor suggestion of your Excellency's most humble servant.

Over the decades, district nurses working in Ireland continued to report on the deplorable conditions of the poor people whom they served, and of the prevalence of sickness among them. One nurse, whose letter was included in the May 1922 edition of the *QNM*, wrote of 'the hundreds who are absolutely starving and insufficiently clothed. I have seen families with nothing in the house but a few potatoes … no milk, tea or flour or means of getting it.' Another gave a truly depressing picture of how 'we have not escaped the still more dreadful scourge of typhus; two whole families have been practically wiped out by the fell disease.' The numbers of nurses did increase, and by September 1935 there were fourteen district nurses in County Galway and a total of forty-five in DNAs stretching from Galway to Kerry, but this was still not adequate to meet the needs of the people.

While London was in the process of professionalising district nursing, a smaller but no less remarkable experiment that had far-reaching consequences was under way in the isolated and neglected village of Gotherington, Gloucestershire. Mrs Elizabeth Malleson (1828–1916), a newcomer to country life, was shocked by the high infant mortality rate and the urgent medical needs of the sick poor in her local hamlet. Described by her daughter, Hope, as having 'the qualities of the pioneer and leader … and the indignant zeal of the reformer', Mrs Malleson was desperate to alleviate the problem, and in 1883 she launched her own campaign to raise funds to pay for a nurse to be trained. Her letters appeared in the Cheltenham press, she canvassed local influential people and produced a graphic prospectus in

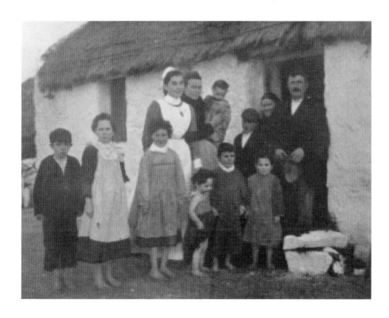

A Lady Dudley Fund district nurse visiting a patient's stone cottage in Ireland (*Queen's Nurses' Magazine*, December 1904).

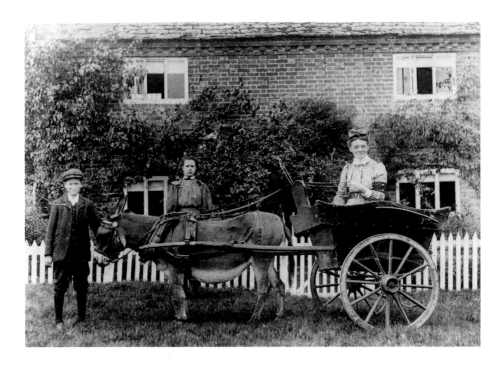

District Nurse
Jenny Wolfe in her
donkey cart at
Gotherington,
Gloucestershire,
c. 1890s.

which she laid bare the situation, writing that 'in village homes there is not even an elementary knowledge of what should be done, and a nurse is urgently needed both to advise and assist, in the mitigation of suffering and the restoration to health.'

In the face of some local opposition, Mrs Malleson secured the support of many doctors and nurses, as well as that of her neighbour, Lady Lucy Hicks-Beach at Winchcombe, whose powerful links and influence helped her realise her ambitious plans. Once established, the rural association went from strength to strength, with the QVJIN playing a very significant part in the growth of this venture. Mrs Malleson, recognising that the national association was concentrating its activities on urban areas, persuaded its council to accept her association as its rural district branch. The QVJIN Rural District branch was constituted in 1888, with county nursing associations established in Hampshire (1891) and Leicestershire (1892).

Life for the rural district nurse was different from that of the urban nurse, as Martha Loane found out when she was sent to her first post, in Buxton, Derbyshire, in 1894. This was one of the Institute's newly affiliated rural branches and covered a district of about 2 square miles with a population of ten thousand. Accommodation was in lodgings of varying comfort. Meals were prepared by the landlady, who sometimes proved to be more of a trial than the patients. Like all Queen's Nurses, the rural district nurse had to maintain her 'Books of Association', which included a case book, as well as a large register of cases and a time book.

Among the patients whom some country district nurses were likely to encounter, not only in the early 1900s but as late as the 1940s, were the hop-pickers, referred to as 'foreigners', who came not from abroad but from villages a few miles or more away. The recollections of one nurse, which appeared in the *QNM* in August 1905, portrayed a 'hopper' woman with rheumatism, who was found 'on straw in a cowshed, with coats for a pillow and bedclothes' and where 'all the cooking had to be done gipsy fashion, in pots slung over a fire in the open'. The most interesting of her patients was a 'hopper' baby with bronchitis, who was living with his eighteen-year-old

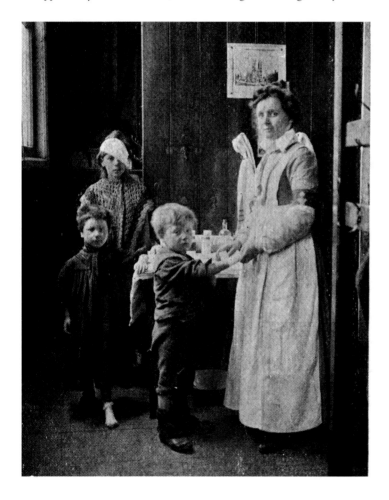

A school nurse in Liverpool, 1905. This was before the formal introduction of a school medical service as a result of the 1907 Education Act.

19

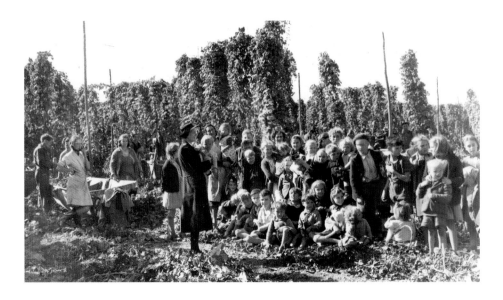

A district nurse/health visitor calls at a Herefordshire hop garden in the 1940s.

mother in the most appalling conditions in a charcoal-burner's tent on the edge of a swamp.

> The doctor told me there was nothing, so I took what would be wanted, and soon had the baby washed and comfortable in a jacket poultice, with pneumonia jacket outside. It had some milk and brandy and went off to sleep.

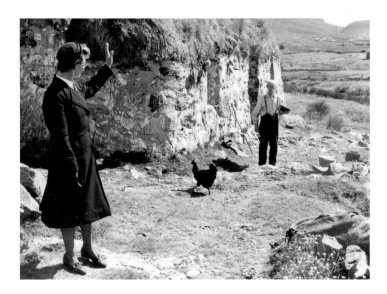

A district nurse calls on a crofter in a remote part of Scotland in the 1950s.

An old man with a cataract benefited from more than her medical expertise, for she made a point of trying to visit in the evening so that she could read to him or listen to his stories of local events long ago. Her care and concern were not taken for granted, for he told her: 'I don't know what I would do without you, and you are as good as a mother to me.'

Another rural district nurse, Nurse Milford, worked in 1910 in a district in Gloucestershire, which had a small population of 1,400, but was spread across an area of approximately 12 square miles, much of which had treacherous roads. Her workload was huge, and in her first year she paid 3,243 visits to 127 medical cases and eighty-six surgical cases, with twenty-seven nights on duty. The five parishes she served proved to be too great a burden for her, and after almost two years in post she reluctantly resigned. The living conditions that the rural district nurse encountered on her rounds remained impoverished into and beyond the 1940s, with visits to travellers living in gipsy caravans, crofters surviving in the remotest parts of Scotland and others whose homes, in the 1950s, lacked indoor sanitation and where water was still being drawn from an outside well.

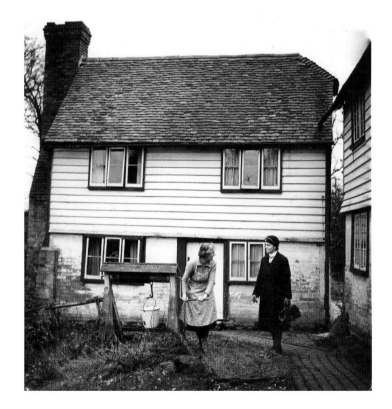

District Nurse Hammond visiting Maude Moarer, who has just become a grandmother twice within three days. Mrs Hammond attends to both babies, c. 1959.' Location uncertain, but probably Brenchley, Kent.

21

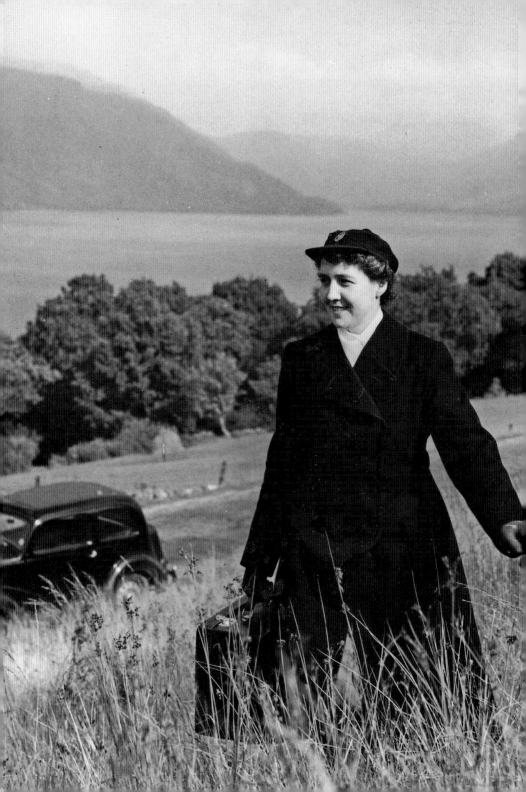

DRESS, EQUIPMENT AND TRANSPORT

FROM THE DAY that the first district nurse set foot on the streets of Liverpool, she was easily recognisable by her outfit of long outdoor cloak and bonnet. But the initial decision of what the Queen's Nurse's uniform of cloak, dress, bonnet and cap should look like had taxed the appointed committee and took a long time to reach. Various designs were discussed and dismissed, and a multitude of fabrics were tried and tested before Queen Victoria finally gave her approval. The resulting ensemble was smart and distinctive, but it was exorbitantly expensive for the time, costing £16 4s. It also featured a badge, an openwork metal reproduction of the royal monogram surmounted by a crown with a surrounding band of the same metal inscribed 'Queen Victoria's Jubilee Institute for Nurses 1887', worn as a pendant on a ribbon or cord around the neck, and a brassard, adorned with the Queen's monogram and worn on the left arm.

To maintain standards, every nurse was provided with a set of instructions that set out precise rules concerning her uniform, and there were watchful eyes around which were quick to point out lapses in the way the district nurse presented herself. Hats were a regular source of comment: one correspondent wrote to the *QNM* in August 1905, at a loss to understand how a country nurse did not know that 'when cycling, a navy blue sailor hat with a blue ribbon is directed to be worn?' Yet another, writing to the magazine's editor in May 1914, chastised a district nurse she encountered at a conference, writing:

> My attention was riveted by the bonnet, the straw of which was almost indiscernible, so caked it was with dirt. The ribbon had faded to the last possible degree, and was broken and frayed. The whole bonnet appeared to be rotting with age... She wore no collar, and the neck of her cloak was greasy and dusty.

With the pedal cycle still supreme, the January 1914 *QNM* recommended district nurses wear a pair of knickerbockers to make cycling more

Opposite:
A district nurse near Loch Fyne, Scotland, in the 1950s.

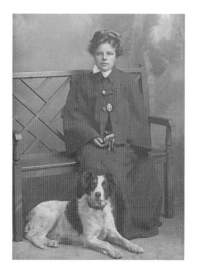

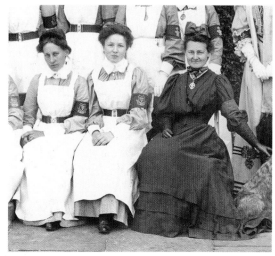

Above: An early
Queen's Nurse
in her outdoor
clothes, 1905.

Above: Queen's Nurses of the Sussex County
Association wearing brassards and badges with
the 'VRI' monogram, 1906.

Left: Figures from a clotihing advertisement in
the *Queen's Nurses' Magazine*, 1913.

Below:
Paper pattern instructions for cycling knickers
(*Queen's Nurses' Magazine*, January 1914).

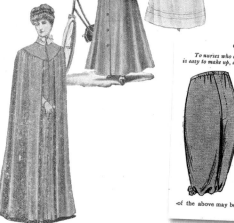

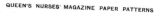

QUEEN'S NURSES' MAGAZINE PAPER PATTERNS.

*To nurses who cycle a good knickerbocker pattern is indispensable. The pattern described here
is easy to make up, and the shape is one which always gives satisfaction to the wearer.*

LADY'S KNICKERS (Weldon pattern 47804).—Suitable for satin, silk,
serge, or Italian cloth. Elastic at waist and knees.

Materials : satin, silk, Italian cloth, fine serge, or alpaca. The
opening at back is quite the latest shape, as by this means much of
the fullness can be dispensed with.

Pattern arranged to suit waist sizes 22, 24, 26, 28, 30 and 34
inches. *Always fit on pattern*, and make any individual alterations
therein before cutting material. Mark material by pattern edges, as
a tacking guide. The notches show how to join the various parts of
this pattern by placing the corresponding notches together.

To CUT : When cutting out allow all turnings and hems on this
pattern. Open out 40-inch material its full width and fold to bring
the two cut edges together ; place knee part of pattern just within
cut edges, and waist towards the fold.

To MAKE : Stitch leg seams, as single notches suggest. Connect
the two legs by stitching seam from front waist downwards, across
top of leg seams, and upwards to within eight or nine inches of back
waist. Turn in and face right side of back opening ; stitch left side
within a wrap of double material. Turn in and hem or face waist
and knees, through slots thus formed insert elastic cut to fit. Button
waist at back.

Quantity of 40-inch material, 1¾ or 2 yards. A Weldon pattern
of the above may be had from 30-32, Southampton Street, Strand, London, post free 7d.

comfortable, and provided full instructions for making this 'indispensable' undergarment. For cycling in the dark, a wide white strap was worn across the shoulder and over the back.

As a matter of convenience, skirt lengths crept up very gradually, and in 1927 the familiar bonnet, floor-length dress and cloak were replaced with a much more modern 'coat-frock' style dress, which was short enough to be hygienic, and far more suited to modern modes of transport, including the motorcar, motorcycle and scooter.

As important for the country district nurse, as advised by Miss Loane as early as July 1904 in *Nursing Notes*, but equally relevant for decades to come, were 'good boots, warm light underwear, stout umbrella and the lightest possible district bag'. The black Gladstone bag became synonymous with the district nurse, and was generally strapped to the carrier of the nurse's bicycle. Made of leather, it had a fitted lining with loops to hold small bottles and jars, and an outside pocket fitted within to accommodate the district nurse's essential instruments. Irene Sankey, recalling her district bag in the 1940s, described it as 'sacrosanct'.

> Never did a piece of equipment receive such loving care! We took soap, towel and nailbrush from the outside pocket, opened the bag, then washed or scrubbed our hands before removing anything from it.

Besides this, there were antiseptic dressings such as lint, gauze and absorbent wool, additional appliances including mackintosh sheeting, water pillows, urinals, an inhaler and a slipper bedpan, none of which was easy to transport by bicycle. Other equipment that the district nurse could obtain for her patients included wheelchairs, rubber water beds, nursing and commode chairs, as well as an extending spinal carriage.

Over the decades, district nurses used every mode of transport available, progressing from the four-legged variety to two-wheeled, then four-wheeled as time went by. In 1890 the district nurse working in rural Gotherington, used a donkey and cart to visit outlying parts of the district. This was such a

New-style clothes illustrated in the *Queen's Nurses' Magazine*, January 1914. 'The coat is cut to give more width across the chest; collar can be worn open or closed. The dress is made in the "coat frock" style with a loose belt.'

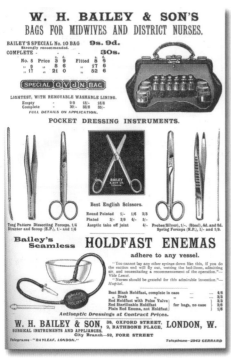

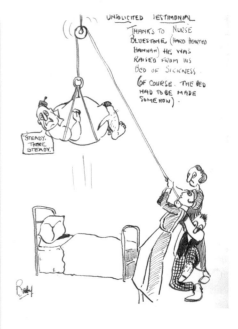

Above: An advertisement for nursing bags and equipment by W. H. Bailey & Sons in the *Queen's Nurses' Magazine*, 1909.

Above right: A patient in Jesmond, Newcastle-upon-Tyne, drew this cartoon of district nurse Elsie Malcolm.

cheap and efficient way of getting around that a second donkey had to be employed. The two donkeys were soon joined by a bicycle, and in 1910 a pony replaced the donkeys, but for many district nurses, from the very early years, the bicycle, and motorised versions of it, was a perennial favourite. But cycling could be very hazardous, and from time to time the

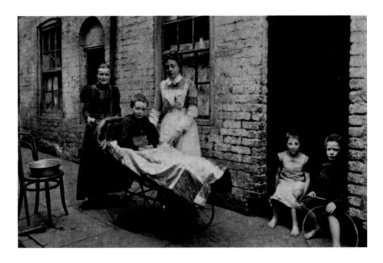

A carriage lent for a tubercular leg case, Liverpool, c. 1905.

QNM reported, with regret, that a district nurse had been involved in a street accident whilst cycling and received fatal injuries.

Even though Mary Stocks recorded a Queen's Nurse on Exmoor still visiting her patients on horseback in the late 1930s, the introduction of various forms of mechanical transport had already transformed life for many district nurses. In 1920, for example, Nurse Radburn of Swanscombe could be seen travelling around her district on a motor scooter. When Nurse Mills joined the Montgomeryshire Nursing Association in 1919, she covered some 12,000 miles of country roads and rough tracks each month by foot, by bicycle and on horseback, only graduating to a motorcycle in 1923, and a car in 1935. Nurse Mills, who was able to boast that she never failed to attend a case, was forced to use a very unusual mode of transport in the winter of 1947, for the only way she could get through the snow drifts was perched on top of a hay load drawn by a caterpillar tractor. Another district nurse, Miss Mary Williams, working in Llandaff, Wales, in 1923, recommended readers of the *QNM* to consider the 'Ivy' motorcycle, which had enabled her to negotiate rough roads and tackle mountainous terrain every day for the past year, in all weathers, 'with only one mishap, namely the snapping of a belt which was righted in a very few minutes'.

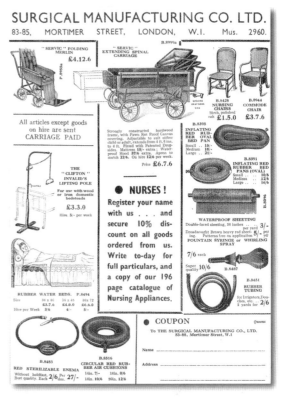

An advertisement for equipment by the Surgical Manufacturing Company Ltd, in the *Queen's Nurses' Magazine*, September 1936.

Travelling was particularly difficult for the district nurse whose patients lived on the many remote islands off the coast of Scotland, for success in reaching them was entirely dependent on the weather. It was not unusual for her, and indeed the doctor, to be ferried on boats manned by local fishermen. One nurse, writing in the *QNM* in November 1925, recalled a frightening three-hour night-time journey across rough seas from Cromore to Stornoway with a sick child on board, certain that they would all be drowned. The same difficulties faced Nurse Donald, the district nurse in Spiddal, a desolate stretch of country on the coast of Ireland, where she had to utilise a variety of 'vehicles' to reach her patients. In August 1905 the

Various means of transport for district nurses; by foot; by horseback in Exmoor; by bicycle in Chipping Campden; by motorcycle; and by car. *Nursing Times,* 19 June 1937.

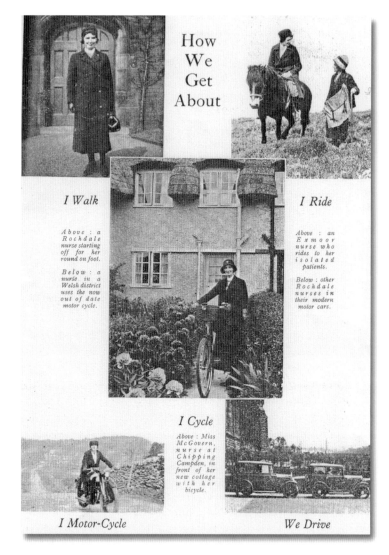

How We Get About

I Walk

Above : a Rochdale nurse starting off for her round on foot.

Below : a nurse in a Welsh district uses the now out of date motor cycle.

I Ride

Above : an Exmoor nurse who rides to her isolated patients.

Below : other Rochdale nurses in their modern motor cars.

I Cycle

Above : Miss McGovern, nurse at Chipping Campden, in front of her new cottage with her bicycle.

I Motor-Cycle

We Drive

An unusual way of getting around in the snow, envisaged in a cartoon drawn by a patient in Jesmond, Newcastle upon Tyne, portraying District Nurse Elsie Malcolm in the 1920s.

7 miles on a bicycle were the easiest part of her journey, for she then had to travel 5 miles on horseback and finally cross a lake in a boat, before reaching the long pathway which led to her patient's house. Not much had changed for these district nurses by 1935, for they had still to be rowed across the water in a curragh to reach some of their patients.

Nothing else came close to the advantages of the motor car, especially for the rural district nurse, for she could cover greater distances, deal with emergencies more quickly and carry more equipment, to say nothing of arriving dry. It soon became the case that if a rural association wanted a nurse they had to offer a car with the post. Nurse Giles, employed in 1940 in a small Somerset district, cherished the Austin Eight car that went with the post, for it enabled her to visit her patients in all weathers in comfort. Irene Sankey was given an ancient second-hand Austin Seven by a member of her DNA around 1940 and, although it was almost falling apart, she could not have managed without it, recalling in 2001:

> That tiny car turned out to be a boon and a blessing, however. It humped along rutted lanes to remote cottages and farmhouses. It kept me dry, but during the winter months it was bitterly cold as there was no heating. I often took a hot water bottle and a rug on my knees. It became a well known sight in Haywards Heath. No-one ever locked their cars in those days and I frequently returned to find a note on the seat, or a bunch of flowers, a half-dozen eggs, a cabbage, a bag of potatoes, a box of chocolates … The note would be signed, but the gifts never bore any names …

I have no trouble in getting round now!

EASY TO RIDE
Cost approx. ½d. per mile
30 MILES PER HOUR
125 MILES PER GALL.
EASILY STORED
Carries Equipment including
"MINNITT"
Gas-Air Apparatus
AT SMALL EXTRA COST

CORGI
Lightweight - Folding
MOTOR CYCLE £43.6.0
plus purchase tax £11.13.10

World Concessionaires—
JACK OLDING & CO. LTD. Telephone: MAYFAIR 5242-3-4
AUDLEY HOUSE · NORTH AUDLEY STREET · LONDON · W.1
(MANUFACTURED BY BROCKHOUSE ENGINEERING [SOUTHPORT] LTD.)

An advertisement for a Corgi motorcycle in the Queen's Nurses' Magazine, 1950.

As more district nurses were employed by individual DNAs, so too did the number of vehicles available. Monica Baly recorded that in 1928 Dorset had six cars and nine motorcycles, but within five years this had increased to twenty-four cars. The DNA in Brighton did not buy their first pair of Morris Eight cars until 1948, but by 1963 the association had a fleet of ten Morris mini-vans, each painted in deep blue and emblazoned with the QN badge and 'Brighton Queen's Nurses Home Nursing Service' in bold white lettering. Not only could the nurses reach the new housing estates that were spread across the district in the most hilly areas, but they were able to carry a wide range of equipment. By 1974, nearly one hundred district nurses were driving the length and breadth of the county, a far cry from 1877 when two nurses tramped the streets of Brighton.

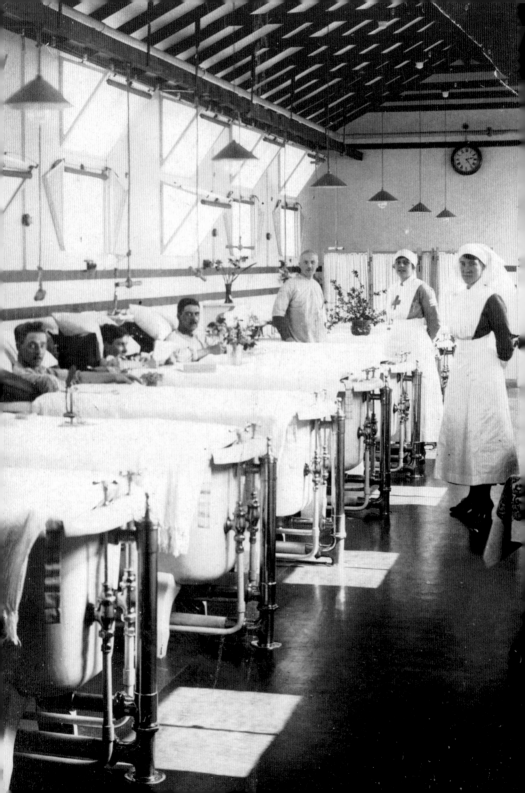

WARTIME: 1914–18

THE DISTRICT NURSE was eminently well qualified to become part of the newly formed Territorial Nursing Service established in 1908 as part of the Territorial Force, specifically to serve in army hospitals in Great Britain and Ireland if the country should be at war. Many QNs had already volunteered for service during the Boer War, and it was not long before their skills were called on again with the outbreak of the First World War in 1914. The district nurses had the full support of the QVJIN and, as the *QNM* wrote in October that year, 'Trained nurses have risen to the emergency, as they always do; they are ready and eager to serve their country in any way that may be demanded of them.' But readers were also reminded that the suffering of war was not confined to soldiers and their families but was felt acutely 'in unemployment, and consequent privation, sickness and general misery in every corner of the land'. Day in and day out, and almost house to house, the district nurse was called upon to counsel, advise and mourn with parents or wives who were suffering loss or separation.

There was an unquantifiable number of hard-working district nurses all over the country who assisted with Red Cross and St John Ambulance work, devoting all their leisure time to this extra role, while still carrying out their usual district duties. Their tasks included giving nursing classes and instructing the Red Cross and St John Ambulance detachments in bandaging, bed-making and splint padding. Miss Mossman in Beaconsfield described superintending the care of convalescent soldiers and sailors housed in what had been the local fever hospital, whilst Miss Tipling from Harrogate described how enthusiastic Red Cross workers were accompanying the district nurses on their rounds so they could become more efficient in 'rendering simple services to the sick'.

Besides this, many district nurses undertook general ward work in the numerous temporary Territorial Hospitals which were set up around the country. Brighton Grammar School, for example, became the Second Eastern General Hospital, where 520 beds in thirty wards were prepared when the

Opposite:
The Gas Ward at Netley Hospital in Hampshire, during the First World War: Patients with mustard gas burns undergo salt bath treatment, 1915. (IWM DRI 33108)

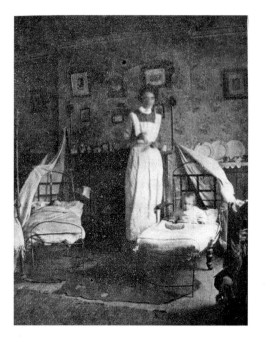

A district nurse on duty, attending patients in their home (*Queen's Nurses' Magazine*, July 1915).

first convoy of three hundred wounded arrived from Mons on 1 September 1914. Here, a quarter or more of the one hundred nurses were QNs. Similarly, in Plymouth, district nurse Miss Tait McKay was acting as Matron at the 520-bed Fourth Southern General Hospital, which comprised the former Salisbury Road Schools and an adjacent church. Seven of the sixty-two nurses were district nurses, and forty of the first batch of 102 'wounded warriors' who arrived 'tired, ill and worn' from the front on 31 August 1914 were stretcher cases. What particularly impressed Miss McKay was the generous response from the public, who provided everything from cigarettes, shaving tackle and gramophones to eggs, fruit and light cakes.

In several districts the nurses were called upon to assist with the medical inspection of Belgian refugees who were given hospitality by their DNA, and in another instance the district nurse was called upon to supervise voluntary workers in a temporary hospital set up to provide medical care for billeted soldiers who had fallen sick. In July 1915 the *QNM* informed readers that district nurses from the Worcester Association were helping nurse sixty-one wounded soldiers at the Battenhall Mount Red Cross hospital. Working alongside members of the Voluntary Aid Detachment, four district nurses were always on duty during the day, and one at night. At Netley, near Southampton, district nurse L. Ethel Nazer found herself treating wounded Sikhs and Gurkhas in the temporary wooden huts that served as a military hospital. She was full of admiration for the bravery of the Gurkhas, whose injuries ranged from hand, arm and shrapnel wounds to heavy stretcher cases and bad frostbite. All the wounds were horribly septic on arrival, and amputations had to be done, but her one consolation was that regular dressings and attention brought very quick improvements. Their efforts were greatly appreciated by the Gurkhas; one, who had lost both eyes, said the 'Sister Sahibs' had been a mother to him and that he would always think of them and pray for them when he got back to India.

Other district nurses, like Miss Maskew, found themselves working on ambulance columns, whose vehicles ranged from Rolls-Royces to small two-seaters. It was her job as Superintendent of the City of London No. 10

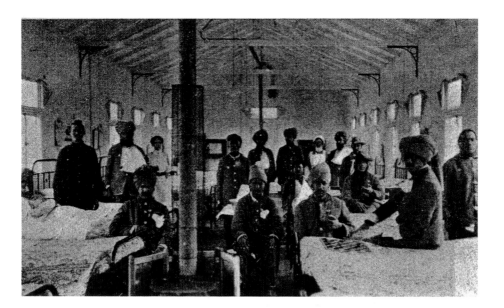

Red Cross Detachment to ensure the safe and comfortable passage of sick and wounded troops from the railway stations to hospital, and she wrote with pride in the *QNM* in April 1916 of how the column had moved 85,000 men since 30 August 1914 without a single death in transit. Her final comments reflected the views of all the district nurses who gave so willingly of their leisure time, for she was 'proud and thankful to be able to do anything for these men who have done so much for us all and who by their cheerfulness and courage have won our undying love and gratitude'.

By January 1916 nearly five hundred district nurses were listed as being on active service, and the *QNM* was a valuable source of information for their counterparts at home, with regular news from nurses in Malta, Serbia, France, Belgium, India and Russia, providing a vivid picture of their experiences, and highlighting their hardiness and resilience. One district nurse, Miss Ethel Ubsdell, went out to France in 1914 with the Society of Friends' Relief Expedition and wrote from Chalons-sur-Marne in April 1915, describing how she had helped rescue a mother and her newborn baby in a nearby village. She could not believe that mother, baby and three other children had survived the bombardment, and the conditions they were living in – vermin-infested rags for clothes, and no food other than a little bread – filled her with despair, relieved only by their rapid recovery once they had been fed and clothed. By October 1915 the intrepid Miss Ubsdell was writing from 'somewhere in France' and

A ward hut at the military hospital at Netley, Hampshire (*Queen's Nurses' Magazine*, January 1915).

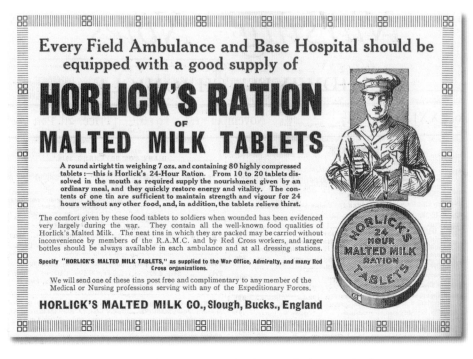

Every Field Ambulance and Base Hospital should be equipped with a good supply of

HORLICK'S RATION
OF
MALTED MILK TABLETS

A round airtight tin weighing 7 ozs. and containing 80 highly compressed tablets :—this is Horlick's 24-Hour Ration. From 10 to 20 tablets dissolved in the mouth as required supply the nourishment given by an ordinary meal, and they quickly restore energy and vitality. The contents of one tin are sufficient to maintain strength and vigour for 24 hours without any other food, and, in addition, the tablets relieve thirst.

The comfort given by these food tablets to soldiers when wounded has been evidenced very largely during the war. They contain all the well-known food qualities of Horlick's Malted Milk. The neat tins in which they are packed may be carried without inconvenience by members of the R.A.M.C. and by Red Cross workers, and larger bottles should be always available in each ambulance and at all dressing stations.

Specify "HORLICK'S MALTED MILK TABLETS," as supplied to the War Office, Admiralty, and many Red Cross organizations.

We will send one of these tins post free and complimentary to any member of the Medical or Nursing professions serving with any of the Expeditionary Forces.

HORLICK'S MALTED MILK CO., Slough, Bucks., England

Advertisers such as Horlicks took advantage of the needs of wounded servicemen (*Nursing Notes*, November 1916).

was working very near the front with the French Flag Nursing Corps. Now she wrote that:

> although we nurse the French soldiers only, we do dressings often for the English Tommies ... We go with the English ambulance right near the trenches sometimes ... and watch the shells bursting over the trenches ... Our hospital is a moving ambulance for clearing cases of infection immediately from the trenches and is therefore bound to be quite near the fighting.

A year later she reported having left Steenvorde and was engaged in 'barge work, going up Nieuport way to bring down wounded and leaving them at hospitals in the interior'.

From Malta, Miss Annie Aspinall, one of several Queen's Nurses working there, wrote of the large number of cases of enteritis and pneumonia that came in every day, and of how, despite being so ill, the surgical patients were 'very good and cheerful, always a smile, and what stories they have to tell of the Dardanelles!'. A letter from Miss M. Rogers, formerly the Superintendent of Hammersmith DNA, writing from Hôpital Temporaire, Arc en Barrois, Haute Marne, France, in October 1916, brought home the

For Wounded Soldiers and all Invalids

When suffering from FEVER induced by illness or the pain of wounds, nothing soothes so much the parched thirst as BARLEY WATER made from

When recovering from the effects of wounds or illness, and Nature wants building up, a basin of GRUEL made nicely from milk and

ROBINSON'S "PATENT" BARLEY

ROBINSON'S "PATENT" GROATS

Recipe for making will be found on every packet and tin.

is always appreciated and works wonders from its strengthening qualities.

KEEN, ROBINSON & CO., LTD., LONDON

reality of being a district nurse on active service. She was on duty every day from seven in the morning to nine at night, and in eight weeks had not had even a half-day off. The only trained nurse, she and her four probationers looked after seventy patients, with sixty to eighty dressings to do every morning. Even though the work was not heavy, it was constant with continual evacuations and intakes, which all meant extra work.

Other district nurses, like Miss Slack in Salonika, were officially prevented from giving details of their work, other than to describe the hospital, made up of tents, and her quarters, which were also under canvas. She was in no doubt that her district work had prepared her very well for this wartime challenge, remarking that 'it is rather like district work in the East End!' This was hardly the case for those district nurses working with the Serbian Relief Fund, for the *QNM* recorded in January 1916 how, having survived a journey menaced continuously by submarines, they had to struggle with the language whilst treating patients with typhus by candlelight. When the nurses later set up a baby clinic and dispensary for the destitute and stricken Serbian mothers, they had the benefit of a pamphlet, 'Hints for Mothers' compiled by Miss Coaling, the superintendent district nurse from Southampton, which was translated into various languages, and printed in Serbian.

Nourishing food for wounded soldiers and invalids, advertised in *Nursing Notes*, January 1917.

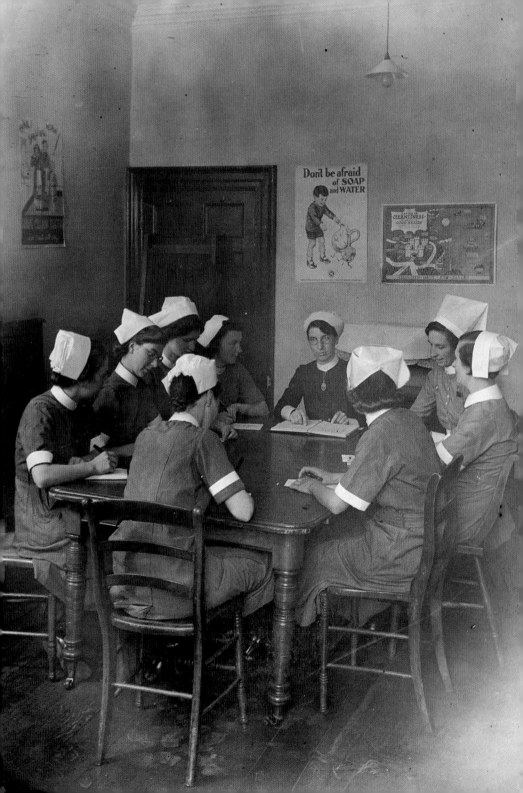

BETWEEN THE WORLD WARS

WHILE THE WAR was still raging abroad, a crisis was looming in the field of district nursing at home, with far fewer women taking up this branch of nursing after completing their hospital training. Miss Watt, Superintendent of Queen's Nurses and Municipal Health Visitors in Motherwell, offered a number of reasons for this in the July 1918 issue of the *QNM*. Many preferred military nursing, with the apparent glamour that surrounded it, and for others the inadequate salaries and extended training were a disincentive. She hoped that when peace came shorter working days would be introduced, easing the burden on the district nurse, but, well before this became a possibility, the pressure on home nursing grew as the country was caught in the grip of the great influenza epidemic. The first case appeared in Glasgow in May 1918, and the virus soon spread to other towns and cities, killing 228,000 people during the next few months, the highest mortality rate for any epidemic since the outbreak of cholera in 1849. The Superintendent of Sheffield DNA, Ellen Hancox, writing in the *QNM* in May 1919, recalled how the first six months of 1918 had been unusually free of illness, but this sense of security was shattered at the end of June, when she and her nurses were faced with an unidentifiable outbreak of serious sickness. September, October and the first week of November, when influenza-related mortality reached its peak, were unforgettable. Her words captured the tragedy of the moment:

> At one time it was only on very rare occasions that we entered a house which had not been visited by the Angel of Death, and we frequently had to superintend the removal of the dead from the bed before we could start nursing the living.

Many patients exhibited symptoms of mania; in others there were abscesses like plague symptoms, and in some cases the eyes swelled and burst, and the patient died after acute suffering. Every death was a tragedy and, besides the numbers of expectant and young mothers who succumbed, young

Opposite:
District nurses meeting with their Superintendent, 1930s.

working people between the ages of eighteen and thirty were the most susceptible and died in most extraordinary numbers. Country districts were not spared the epidemic, and the burden on the local district nurses was especially heavy. In a very hilly district in Yorkshire, for example, during November and the early part of December 1918, two solitary district nurses treated 116 influenza patients, and in one week alone made 306 visits.

The Armistice, signed on 11 November 1918, brought peace, but there was no let-up in the demands on the district nurse and, despite hopes of attracting more women into the profession, the staff shortages continued. Monica Baly records that ten district nurses died as a result of influenza in 1919, 324 resigned but only 121 new nurses were placed on the roll. The London DNA hit upon a solution in August 1919 by setting up the London Emergency Nurses' Register, appealing to women to offer their professional services on a temporary basis, to cover, for example, holidays and periods of epidemics such as measles, whooping cough and influenza 'when a sufficiency of nurses would save many precious lives.'

Meanwhile, the day-to-day routine of the district nurses continued much as it had in late 1890s Liverpool. On a typical morning, in towns and cities up and down the country, they would have breakfast at eight o'clock, then fill their bags with all the necessary equipment, lotions and potions before leaving the Central Home for their first round of patients. Back at the Home between 1.00 and 1.30 p.m. for dinner, they would then report any new cases or changes in the condition of any patients to the Superintendent,

District nurses preparing to leave their home to go on their rounds, 1950s.

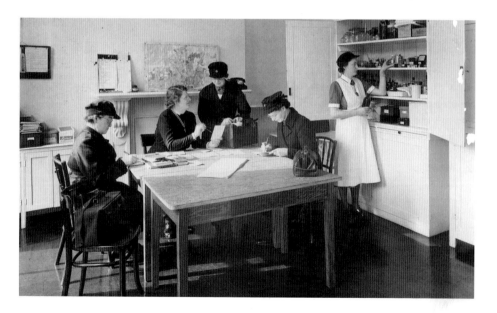

before going off duty for two hours. Returning to work after tea, the district nurse had a three-hour evening round, making sure that all her patients were comfortable for the night. Only then could she go back to the Central Home for supper. But the day's work was far from finished, for reports had to be made, case and time books completed, and equipment cleaned and prepared for the next day, to say nothing of the occasional emergency call.

Any spare time might be spent glancing through the pages of the *QNM*, which remained a valuable source of information for district nurses. There were, for example, helpful hints on cooking and invalid recipes, which included junket, considered a good standby, as it was quick to make and appealed to children if it was sprinkled with chocolate. Other delicacies designed to appeal to the sick were hot potato dogs – a cored potato, stuffed with sausage meat and baked in the oven – and a country chop suey. Probationers found the magazine especially useful in preparing for their examinations, as issues regularly included sample questions such as this, published on 17 September 1914: 'If sent to attend an urgent operation for strangulated hernia, how would you prepare the patient and the room?' Three years later, in March 1917, the following question was typical of those being posed: 'If it were considered necessary to sterilise milk supplied from a dairy how would you do it? What diseases may be conveyed by milk?' This serves as a reminder of the real danger of contracting tuberculosis from unpasteurised milk and was an issue that the district nurses in Brighton learnt to deal with in the 1930s, thanks to their local doctor, Neville Cox. He taught them the value of tuberculin injections and impressed upon them the importance of sterilising syringes by boiling before and after use.

As a report published in *Town and Country News* in West Sussex in June 1934 made clear, general nursing and midwifery were only part of the job, for the district nurses, here as elsewhere, undertook all public health duties, including that of school nurse. This was not a new role, but the demands had certainly increased since 1904 when the Education Committee in Widnes first appointed a district

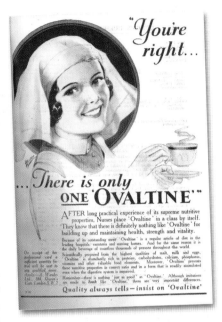

An advertisement for Ovaltine in the *Queen's Nurses' Magazine*, 1935.

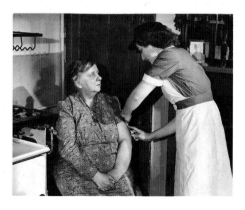

A district nurse gives a patient medication by injection, c. 1949.

District Nurse
Catriona MacAskill
weighing a baby in
a net bag, 1950s.

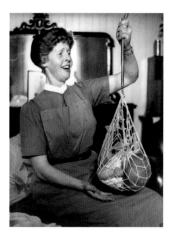

nurse to 'attend to the minor ailments of children, both for their sakes as a curative and preventive measure, and also to secure a higher attendance'. Many more district nurses took up this new opportunity after the 1907 Education (Administrative Provisions) Act introduced a school medical service, and Liverpool, the cradle of district nursing, was once again in the vanguard of social progress, for in 1909 two of the nurses on ordinary district work attended a school for one day a week.

What the district
nurse wore in
1936 (*Queen's
Nurses' Magazine,*
June 1936).

Elsewhere, Gloucestershire County Council paid 1s 0d an hour for the attendance of a Queen's Nurse in school, whilst Tunbridge Wells went even further and paid £100 a year for the full-time service of a Queen's school nurse. The East London Society's nurses were not far behind, for they began to attend the School Centre in Poplar in 1912.

School nursing was also in its infancy in Irish national schools and, according to an anonymous district nurse writing in the *QNM* on 31 August 1909, the scheme 'must prove of the greatest advantage in checking disease of different kinds amongst children', which included accidents, burns, eczema and warts, as well as the highly contagious ringworm and impetigo. For the children in West Sussex in 1934 the school clinic offered the opportunity of them

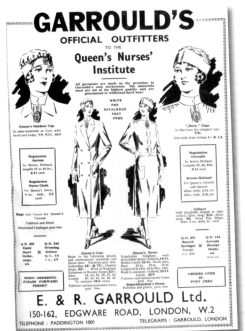

seeing familiar faces around … and the mother possesses the assurance that her treasure will be safe with her own district nurse. Foster-children, nurse-children, boarded-out children, all come under her care, and their home conditions are regularly reviewed.

The district nurse was especially popular with children, and this was poignantly demonstrated in the entries for a children's essay competition held in Holbeck, Leeds, in June 1939, as reported in the *QNM*. One child wrote:

> District nurses go to your house because they want you to get better. They
> are kind to you and they are healthy and strong … One day a district nurse
> came to me when I had rheumatism and measles. I like the district nurse
> very much indeed. She would tell me stories when my brothers were at
> school and my mother at the workshop.

Another child commented: 'She has not to be lazy or slow. She is always ready. She passes a hard test to be a district nurse.'

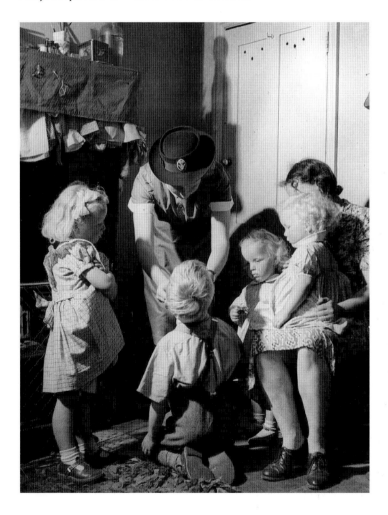

Nurse Jeal visiting
a child at home
with tonsillitis.

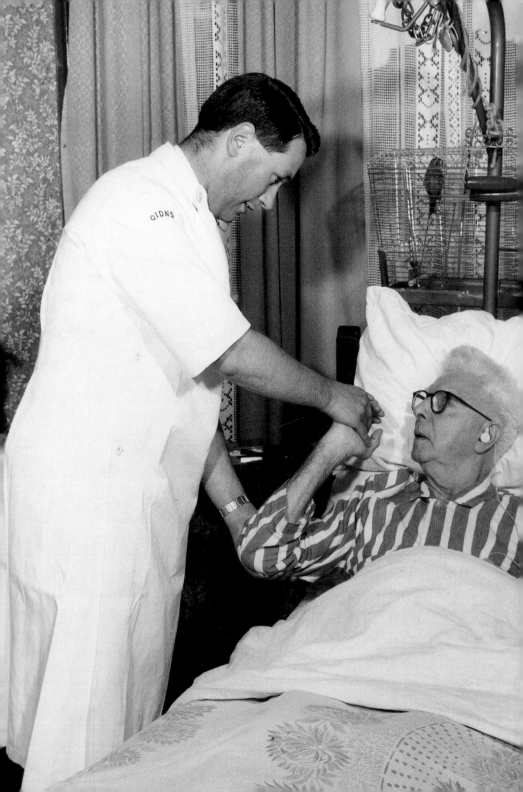

WARTIME, THE NATIONAL HEALTH SERVICE AND BEYOND

THE DISTRICT NURSE was again called upon to contribute to the war effort during the Second World War, particularly on the Home Front. In case any nurse doubted the value of her contribution, the *QNM* assured them that every nurse was 'vitally necessary to their hard-working brothers and sisters who are providing "the sinews of war"'. For their personal safety, each nurse was immediately issued with a tin hat and a service gas-mask, which was a superior model to the one used by civilians. A new uniform regulation had also to be strictly observed, and the sight of the district nurse wearing a wide white strap across one shoulder and over the back became commonplace. Some DNAs, such as Bagley Wood, near Oxford, also provided a staff air-raid shelter. As well as the new uniform arrangements, there were the limitations of clothes rationing to contend with, and travelling around the district became more difficult as autocycles and mechanised cycles were banned during the black-out. But this was a minor inconvenience when compared to the dangers faced by the district nurses working on the remote islands in the Atlantic and the North Sea, who, by 1941, had the use of small aeroplanes to enable them, and the doctors, to travel from island to island.

In the early part of the war, one of the country district nurse's roles was to meet evacuees, mothers and children, from London and other cities at railway stations. She was also responsible for carrying out health checks before the youngsters were billeted, and in January 1940 the district nurses in Bagley Wood had the dubious task of making four hundred visits to the specially established clinic to undertake head-lice inspections. Being among the civilians in the front line of battle, the nurse needed to boost morale and to allay fear and panic during enemy air attacks, but it was not long before the air raids impacted on the district nurses' work; many nurses' homes were destroyed by bombs, as in Coventry during 1940, and some nurses were killed.

Despite these losses, the bravery of nurses became renowned, with instances being recorded in the pages of the issues of the *QNM* (now

Opposite:
A male district
nurse visiting
a patient, 1967.

significantly thinner as a result of paper rationing). One account, in the December 1940 publication, vividly captured the experience of the Blitz on east London on 7 September 1940:

> The noise, the whistling, the crashing of the bombs was alarming. Passers-by were glad to almost fall into our Home and along to our shelter. Our dining-room was complete with sand bags and other protection, and there we led them. Only two of the nursing staff were in the Home, others were all out on their districts, for it was but 3 p.m. We sheltered for an hour, perhaps a little longer. The house trembled, and with some crashes we felt that the front had gone. We heard the noise of falling buildings, the terrible crackling of the fires, and the unmistakeable smell of smoke … We bring in the homeless and shocked ones, and attend to them, and as soon as it is light, various members of the staff set off for the schools and church halls to help tend and feed the homeless … Tragic are the happenings when new blocks of flats are hit … invariably the trench shelters are wrecked and the walls cave in. Twenty hours, and the rescue squads still digging. One hundred and seventy in the shelter, and all brought out alive but six. The last man, still conscious, and the doctor is near to give morphia. 'No, thank you, doc; just a cup of tea, thanks.'

The heroism of the district nurses in the city of Plymouth, which was severely damaged when it came under fire in March and April 1941, was commended by the *Western Morning News*, which reported how they thought nothing of picking their way across debris to reach a patient's house, or of arriving at a home during a raid to find, as Miss McCarthy did, three incendiary bombs blazing in it. Before attending to the sick person, she extinguished the bombs with the help of an elderly man, and then went on with her business as usual. The only concession made to 'womanly fears' was that, instead of one, two or three nurses went out together to answer calls for aid.

Miss Cantrill and Miss McCarthy picking their way across debris left by an air raid to reach the house of a patient (*Queen's Nurses' Magazine*, September 1941).

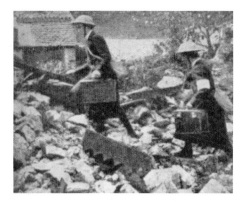

Less dangerous was the ministering role played by district nurses, for they often found themselves serving the sick in the centres that were set up in cities for those who had been bombed out of their homes. Miss Edwards, a Queen's Nurse, reported from one provincial city in January 1942 that, following an air raid, several hundred people were taken to the centre and 'found hot drinks being prepared, hot-water bottles being put into beds and a band of willing helpers giving mothers a hand

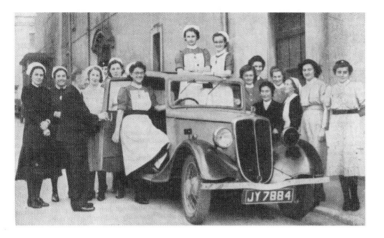

Nurses of the Three Towns (Plymouth) Nursing Association (*Queen's Nurses' Magazine*, December 1944).

with large families'. The comfort and reassurance that these frightened people derived from seeing the familiar district nurse to help them through their worst experience was priceless. Nurse Edwards was certainly humbled, writing: 'Their gratitude was pathetic – it was impossible to impress upon them how honoured we were to serve them.'

This same devotion to duty was evident amongst nurses who worked abroad, as a personal account published in the *QNM* in September 1940 showed. The unnamed author was serving with Queen Alexandra's Imperial Military Nursing Service in a French port and recalled:

The *Queen's Nurses' Magazine* promoting an Ambulance Fund, September 1940.

When winter came there was much sickness among the troops and also unfortunately among the staff ... One great drawback to this hospital was no hot-water system ... everything had to be managed on one very poor gas ring and very 'tricky' Primus stove ... When hostilities began in real earnest, and people from all over the place were coming through our port after the evacuation of Dunkirk, we had to become a casualty clearing station instead of a base hospital, and send cases fit to travel straight back to England. Several hundred sisters came to our hospital for the night on their way home. Many had lost all their kit. Some whom I knew personally had lost their hospital ship; it went down at Dunkirk. They were thankful for a mattress on the floor to sleep on after many days and nights of harassing experiences.

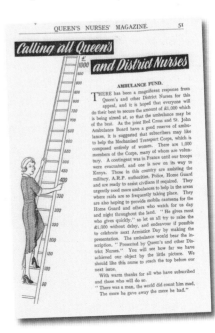

With clothes rationing in force until March 1949, the Austerity Dress used less material than earlier designs.

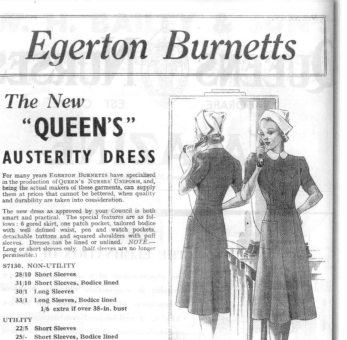

Egerton Burnetts

The New "QUEEN'S" AUSTERITY DRESS

For many years EGERTON BURNETTS have specialised in the production of QUEEN'S NURSES' UNIFORM, and, being the actual makers of these garments, can supply them at prices that cannot be bettered, when quality and durability are taken into consideration.

The new dress as approved by your Council is both smart and practical. The special features are as follows : 6 gored skirt, one patch pocket, tailored bodice with well defined waist, pen and watch pockets, detachable buttons and squared shoulders with puff sleeves. Dresses can be lined or unlined. *NOTE.—* Long or short sleeves only (half sleeves are no longer permissible.)

S7130. NON-UTILITY
28/10 Short Sleeves
31/10 Short Sleeves, Bodice lined
30/1   Long Sleeves
33/1   Long Sleeves, Bodice lined
    1/6 extra if over 38-in. bust

UTILITY
22/5   Short Sleeves
25/-   Short Sleeves, Bodice lined
23/6   Long Sleeves
26/1   Long Sleeves, Bodice lined
    1/3 extra if over 38in. bust

All prices include one White Detachable Collar.

Write for our fully illustrated Price List with patterns of the actual materials, sent Post Free on receipt of 1 penny. Prices subject to alteration without notification.

EGERTON BURNETTS LTD. QN. Dept., WELLINGTON, SOMERSET
London Branch
EGERTON BURNETTS LTD. 30 BUCKINGHAM PALACE ROAD, S.W.1
TELEPHONES : WELLINGTON 4.   VICTORIA 7082

Contractors to the " Queen's " Insitute of District Nursing and many County Nursing Associations ; appointed by the General Nursing Councils for England and Wales, and Scotland, to supply Registered Nurses' Uniforms, etc. Officially appointed Makers of Uniform for Queen Alexandra's Imperial Military Nursing Service.
Carriage and C.O.D. charges paid on orders of 40/- in the British Isles.

Alongside those undertaking war-related nursing was a small army of district nurses who, like Nurse Irene Sankey, performed a multiple role in the community, as she described:

> The district nurse, the midwife and the health visitor were one and the same – three in one, so to speak. As the midwife I would say 'goodbye' to a new mother on the fourteenth day and as the health visitor greet her 'good morning' on the fifteenth. The patients appreciated the continuity of care …

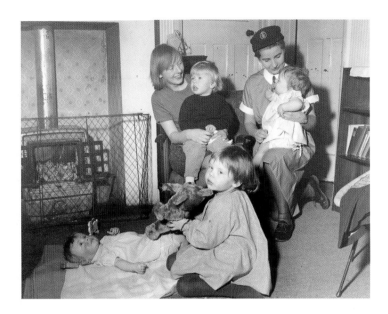

Post-vaccination visit by the district nurse, as health visitor, c. 1950s.

Patients in Leicester welcomed four young male nurses, who began training with the Queen's Institute in 1947. Until then, district nursing was

Queen's Nurse Geoff Hunt by his 1938 Morris Eight, c. 1963.

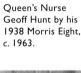

traditionally a woman's job, but the experiment proved successful and before long more male nurses put themselves forward as Queen's candidates. One pioneer, Mr Gillett, recalled his training, which was very different from that followed by his female counterparts half a century earlier:

> [I] was surprised to find how comprehensive and wide the educational syllabus is. I thoroughly enjoyed my lectures and visits. The lectures included medicine, hygiene, child welfare and management, poor law, charitable societies, local government, diet and Health Insurance, among many others. Visits were made to a dairy where the pasteurisation processes were in progress, to the city sewage works, a Mental Deficiency Home, a Nursery School, a School Clinic, a Child and Maternity Clinic, a large factory (where we were conducted round by an Industrial Nurse), and a Psychiatry Clinic. These were just a few of our varied visits. A complete half day was spent with a Health Visitor.

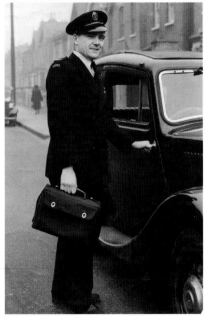

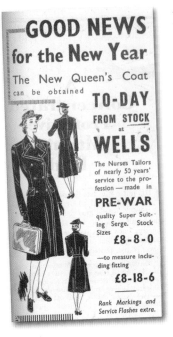

An advertisement for an outdoor coat in the *Queen's Nurses' Magazine*, 1947. L. Wells & Company claimed to be 'the nurses' tailors', with fifty-three years of service to the profession.

As he was permitted to nurse only men, he was given responsibility for all the male patients across the district, which surprised some people as there were many difficult female cases on the books. In an average day he travelled about 21 miles, apparently by bicycle. When district nurse Geoff Hunt moved to Eastbourne in 1953, tuberculosis was still a killer disease, and he had no doubt that home nursing played a huge part in bringing about a sea change in the occurrence of pulmonary tuberculosis in Great Britain:

The disease had almost reached epidemic proportions by the time we rolled up our sleeves, donned our gowns, put our bags on those sheets of newspaper, boiled our syringes and needles and slipped the 5ml dose into the patient's rear end. Thousands of us, treating maybe four to eight patients each day. Nice to know we helped to change History in such a significant way, isn't it?

By then, the National Health Service (NHS), introduced in 1948, had transformed the way district nursing was provided, for it became a state scheme, paid for through National Insurance contributions, and was made available by local health authorities. Gone were the days of fund-raising, house-to-house collections, donations and subscriptions, for now anyone who required home nursing,

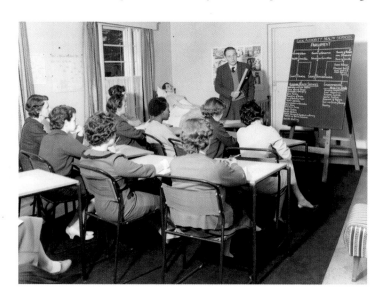

Nurses undergoing training in 1950. Here they are learning about the structure of the National Health Service.

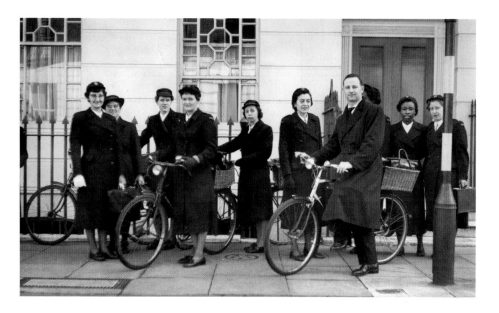

regardless of their financial circumstances, could receive the services of the district nurse free of charge. As far as Nurse Irene Sankey was concerned, this was a red-letter day, for she had found asking for money 'embarrassing and distasteful, asking them about their income and expenditure':

District nurses leaving the nurses' home on their bicycles, 1950s.

> This information, together with other details necessary in our Case Book, was taken to the Superintendent who decided how much they should contribute, the amount varying from as little as threepence to as much as two and six per week or per visit, depending on individual circumstances. The 'necessitous poor' was [sic] nursed free of charge. Monday was pay-day. We went out with our tiny receipt books and most of us had a small tin for the money …

A district nurse and a general practitioner confer while on their rounds, 1959.

Other nurses, such as Nurse Evans in Llanfair Caereinion, Wales, identified different positive aspects, for every case could now have a nurse and doctor if required. One of the greatest aids to communication, as far as she was concerned, was the telephone, for she could get speedy help for the seriously ill and summon a doctor at very short notice. There was also the benefit of a new mobile emergency squad within

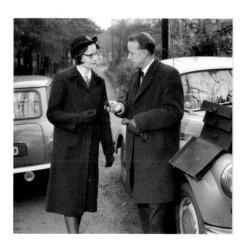

Queen's Nurse
Parsons measuring
a child on a school
visit, 1949.

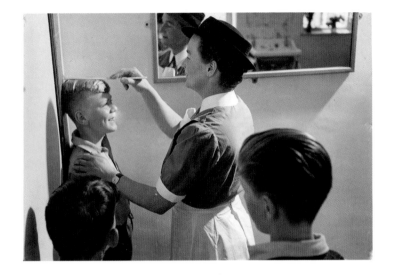

30 miles of her. By the 1950s the days of a single telephone in a village were gone as public kiosks became commonplace and telephones were installed in private houses and district nurses' homes. For a district nurse working from home in a Lancashire town in 1960, this was a mixed blessing, as she found herself delayed in the mornings, having to answer innumerable calls. Yet another modern invention, the car radio telephone, which became available in the late 1960s, made instant communication possible. Far less sophisticated was a tried and tested method of locating the nurse during the day, available

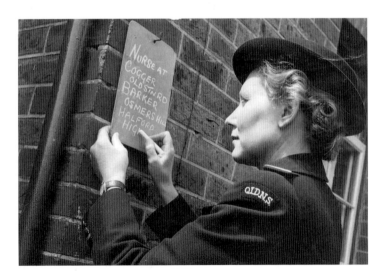

District Nurse
Dorothy Jeal
leaving details
of where she had
gone on a slate
outside her home
in 1949. People
needed to know
how to find her
in an emergency.

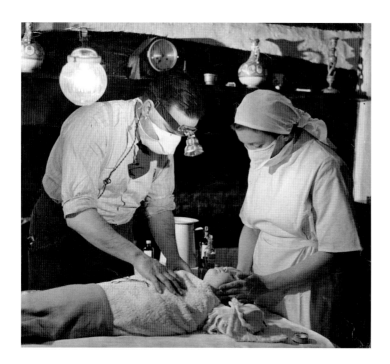

A nurse aids a doctor performing a tracheotomy on a child with diphtheria in a house in the 1950s.

to anyone who called at her house, for there, fixed outside for all to see, was a slate noticeboard with a list of the day's calls, names and addresses, chalked on it.

As a way of introducing the public to the district nurse, and to encourage people to join their local DNA, a number of films were made for the cinema, which showed nurses carrying out their day-to-day duties. The first of these was produced in the early 1930s, but it was a 1952 black and white film, *District Nurse*, featuring Queen's Nurses Dorothy Jeal and Nora Parsons that captivated audiences and gave a real insight into the invaluable place of the district nurse in the modern community. A typical day for them included calls to patients in their homes (including a houseboat) in the village of Wadhurst, Sussex, and the surrounding countryside, attending the local schools and holding infant welfare clinics. Besides this, the nurse acted as

Record cards for district nurses, *District Nursing*, July 1958.

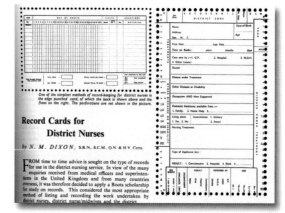

a social worker, organising chiropody and home help, visited hospitals to discuss a patient's convalescence with the nursing sister, gave sex education lessons to schoolgirls, ante-natal tuition to expectant mothers, and had, on rare occasions, to assist the doctor in performing life-saving surgery in a patient's home when an emergency arose. This was a real test of her competence for it required prompt action and resourcefulness to adapt to makeshift conditions in a cool, calm way. Although many nurses said they needed to have a mind like a card index, precise record keeping was vital and, instead of the books kept by the early-twentieth-century nurses, Nurse Jeal and her peers had specially printed cards to complete, stored so they were readily available for reference.

Maintaining standards was equally important, and the district nurse in the 1950s was supervised in much the same way as her predecessors had been in the late nineteenth century. Inspections sometimes revealed failings in local areas, as in Blackpool, where not enough late visits were being made to patients, mainly because there was no rota for evening visits or emergency calls. As always, district nurses worked with and under the

A district nurse/midwife with a class of expectant mothers, 1960s.

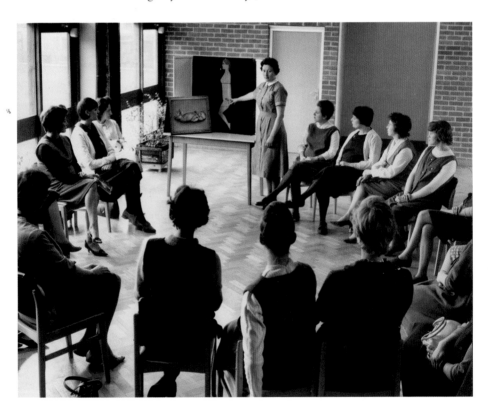

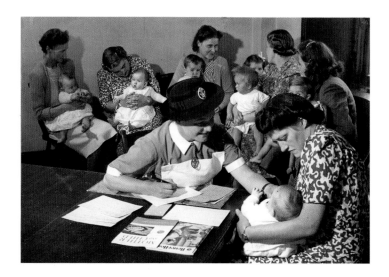

District Nurse Nora Parsons at an infant welfare clinic in the 1950s.

direction of the doctor, often accompanying him or her on their rounds, but a new development was for nurses to be in contact with or attached to the general practitioner's healthcare centre. This was the situation that Dorothea Beatty found herself in in 1953, when she was appointed to work at the very first purpose-built health centre in Scotland, at Sighthill in Edinburgh. Recounting her experiences in *District Nursing* in October 1960, she wrote of being quite unprepared for the contrast between the conditions she was used to and this state-of-the-art clinic, with its contemporary furnishings, private examination rooms and inviting waiting rooms, to say nothing of the modern treatment rooms complete with autoclave and large sterilisers. Her description captured the very essence of the NHS, for the aim of the centre was 'to draw the various health services closer together and enable them to co-operate for the benefit of the patient in the prevention and treatment of ill health, both mental and physical'. Summing up the keynote of her work, she concluded that it 'must surely be co-operation day by day with the large team of workers who were hoping to provide improved family health services'.

Having secured a place in society, the district nurse in twenty-first century Britain is still very much a part of the community and continues to provide care in people's homes. The advent of modern technology and medical advances have had an impact on the nature and administration of care, and their job now includes team management and more complex patient assessments, especially for those with long-term conditions. But a fundamental part of the work begun by William Rathbone is still to promote healthy lifestyles and provide health education. More than ten

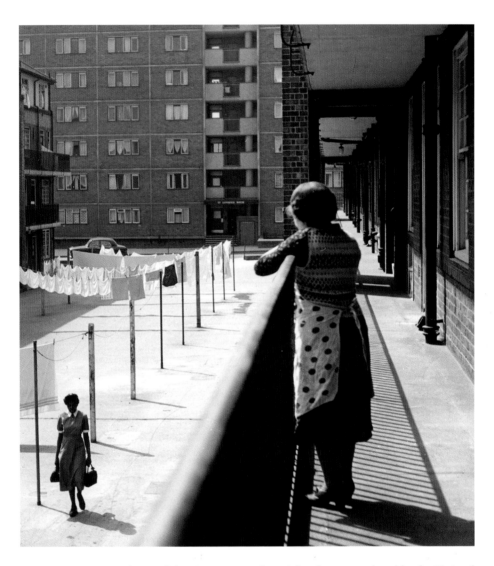

A district nurse visiting a patient on a council estate in the 1960s.

thousand district nurses, male and female, are employed by the National Health Service to provide patients and their families with emotional help and advice, and to teach basic care-giving skills where needed. In this respect, Florence Nightingale's description of the role of the district nurse, which was 'to raise the homes of your patients so they never fall back again into dirt and disorder', resonates today, notwithstanding the progress of modern medicine to treat and cure diseases that were unrecognised in the 1880s.

FURTHER READING

Baly, Monica. *A History of the Queen's Nursing Institute. 100 Years 1887–1987.* Croom Helm, 1987.

Beatty, Dorothea. 'On the Internal Phone', *District Nursing*, October 1960, pp. 154–5.

Cotterill, Edith. *Nurse on Call. Tales of a Black Country District Nurse.* Century Hutchinson, 1986.

Dingwall, R., Rafferty, A. M., and Webster, Charles (editors). *An Introduction to the Social History of Nursing.* Routledge, 1988. Includes historical information about district nursing.

Evans, David Mills. *A District Nurse in Rural Wales before the National Health Service.* Gwasg Carreg Gwalch, 2003.

Gill, Maud F. *District Nursing in Brighton 1877–1974.* Benedict Press, Brighton, 1974.

Howse, Carrie. *Rural District Nursing in Gloucestershire 1880 – 1925.* Reardon, Cheltenham, 2008.

Markham, Joan. *My Little Black Bag.* Robert Hale, 1973. A recollection of district nursing in Lancashire *c*. 1950.

Stocks, Mary. *A Hundred Years of District Nursing.* George Allen & Unwin, 1960.

The Annual Reports of the Borough of Portsmouth Association for Nursing the Sick Poor (1885–1939) are held in the Local Collection at Portsmouth Central Library, ref 610.6.

The papers of the QVJIN, and other district nursing-related material, can be found in the Wellcome Institute Library and Contemporary Medical Archives, London.

A Google search reveals the existence of documents in the National Archive and Public Record Offices relating to local District Nursing Associations all over the United Kingdom, providing evidence of their work. Few appear to have been written up.

National Archives, Kew. PRO 30/63 Records of the Queen's Institute of District Nursing, covering dates from 1850 to 1949, with papers from all associations preserved to 1914. Thereafter, only county and selected urban and rural areas are preserved.

A Friend of the Family. District Nursing in Twentieth Century Britain 1859–2009 (a DVD), can be obtained direct from the Queen's Nursing Institute, 3 Albemarle Way, London EC1V 4RQ, or from the online shop at www.districtnursing150.org.uk This website celebrates the 150th anniversary in 2009 of the foundation of district nursing in Liverpool, and is an excellent source of information.

INDEX